MR.
LANCI
TALKS MENTAL HEALTH

DISCLAIMER

I, Vincent A. Lanci, am not a medical professional and all content found in this book, *Mr. Lanci Talks Mental Health*, is for informational purposes only.

The content in this book, *Mr. Lanci Talks Mental Health*, is not intended to be a substitute for professional medical advice, treatment, or diagnosis.

Always seek the advice of qualified individuals, including your physician or contacting healthcare providers, with any inquiries related to a medical condition.

Never delay or disregard seeking professional medical advice because of something you have read in this book, *Mr. Lanci Talks Mental Health*.

Illustrated by Chris Helene Bridge
Designed by Marla Yadira Garcia

MR.
LANCI
TALKS MENTAL HEALTH

VITAL INFORMATION
FOR AN OPTIMAL MINDSET

VINCENT A. LANCI

ACKNOWLEDGMENTS

My family for their continued support.

Dr. Denise McDermott for being an incredible friend, mental wellness influencer, and role model for all.

Chris Helene Bridge for the illustrations, guidance, and conversations during the creation of this book.

Rod Buchen for the continued mentorship and friendship since my first day of graduate school.

…and **YOU!** Yes, you; reading this book!
Thank you for making your mental health a priority.

Table of Contents

Preface.. 6

DAY 1
Listening to Your Body............................ 8
with Dr. Richard Boccio

DAY 2
Self-Expression and Gratitude 14
with Ms. Chris Helene Bridge

DAY 3
Living a Healthy Lifestyle......................... 20
with Mr. Jon Infeld

DAY 4
Love and Care... 26
with Dr. Denise McDermott

DAY 5
Yoga, Meditation, and Spirituality 32
with Mr. Tony Alexander

DAY 6
Socializing and Support 38
with Mr. James Durand

DAY 7
Rest and Breaks.. 44
with Mr. Vincent A. Lanci

How They Met.. 50

Works Cited 51

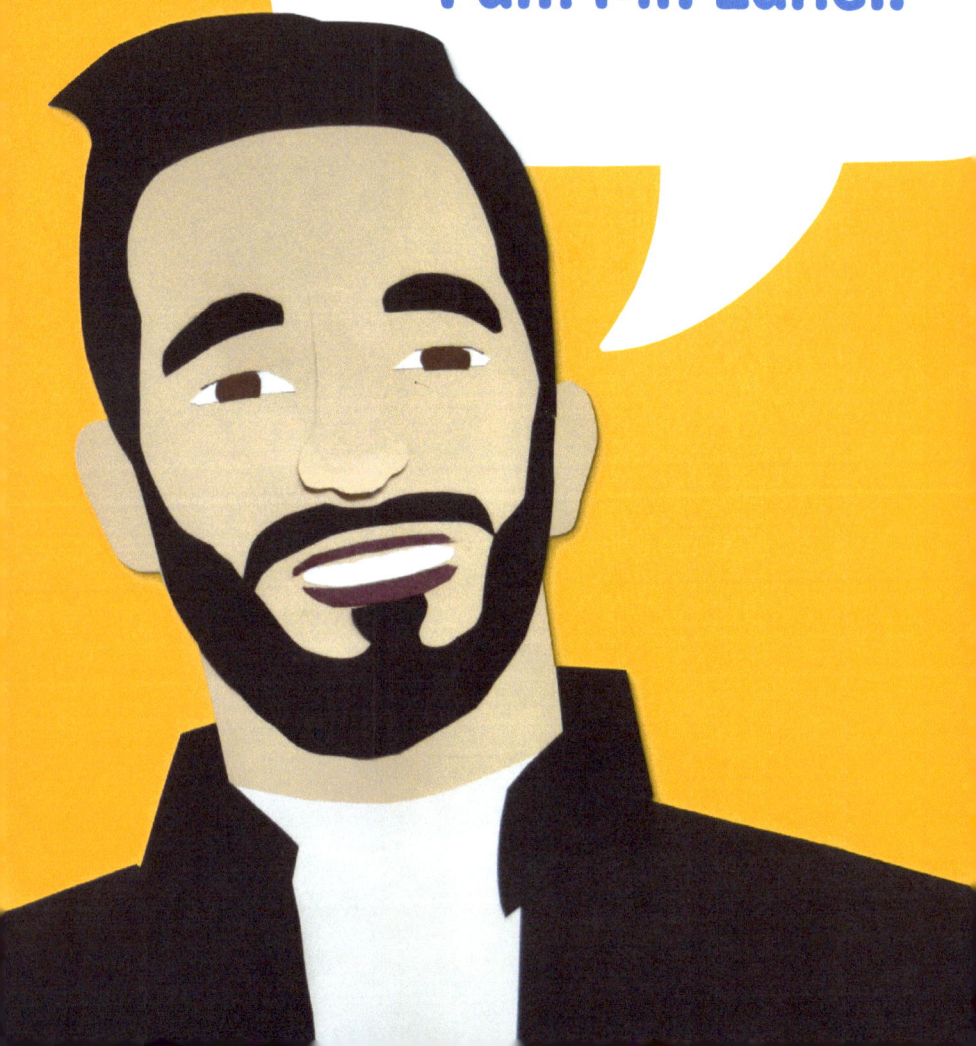

This resource contains information you may not know that will help you feel your best!

This resource contains information you may not know that will help you feel your best!

When I was 21 years old, I was the victim of a hit-and-run accident. At first, there was speculation from the doctors as to whether I would make it through the initial night. As I remained alive, their concerns switched to whether I would ever be able to go to the bathroom on my own, walk, or talk properly again.

Over time, I began recovering from this horrific event, and quickly learned that I needed to make my mental health a priority. I want to help you do the same by focusing on improving your mental health one day at a time for one week.

Join me and some of my favorite health experts in learning some tips that are sure to make a difference in anyone's life!

To visit Vincent A. Lanci's website, visit:
https://www.VincentALanci.com

To listen to Vincent A. Lanci's song *Mental Health Wealth*, visit:
https://www.soundcloud.com/VincentALanci

To purchase Vincent A. Lanci's first book,
Left for Dead: A Story of Redemption, visit:
https://www.VincentALanci.com

To purchase Vincent A. Lanci's second book,
How to Transform Your Mindset When the Norm is Changed, visit:
https://www.VincentALanci.com

To listen to Vincent A. Lanci's *A Mental Health Break Podcast*, visit:
https://amentalhealthbreak.buzzsprout.com

To listen to Vincent A. Lanci's *That Entrepreneur Show*, visit:
https://thatentrepreneurshow.buzzsprout.com

Day 1

LISTENING TO YOUR BODY

with

Dr. Richard Boccio

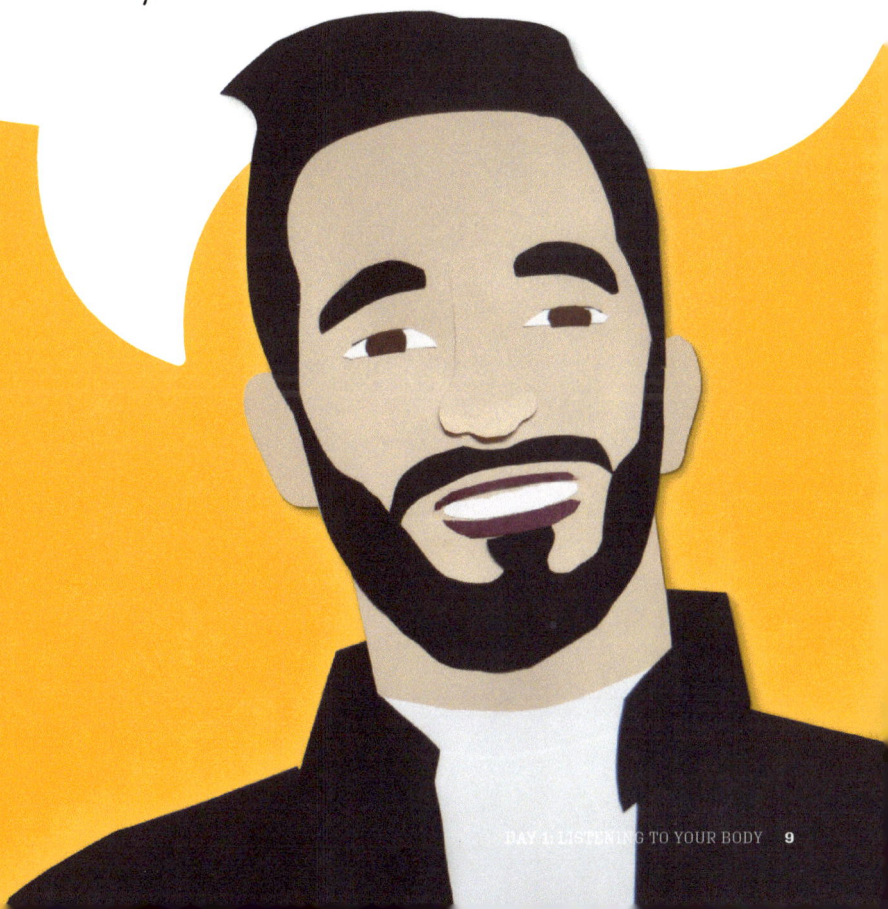

Mr. Lanci Says

1. Your physical AND mental health need care

2. Listen to what your body is telling you

3. Use your senses

Meet the Expert

Dr. Richard Boccio is an Emergency Medicine Resident Physician in Miami, Florida. He graduated with honors from The Ross University School of Medicine. Dr. Boccio is dedicated to helping people reach peak mental and physical health.

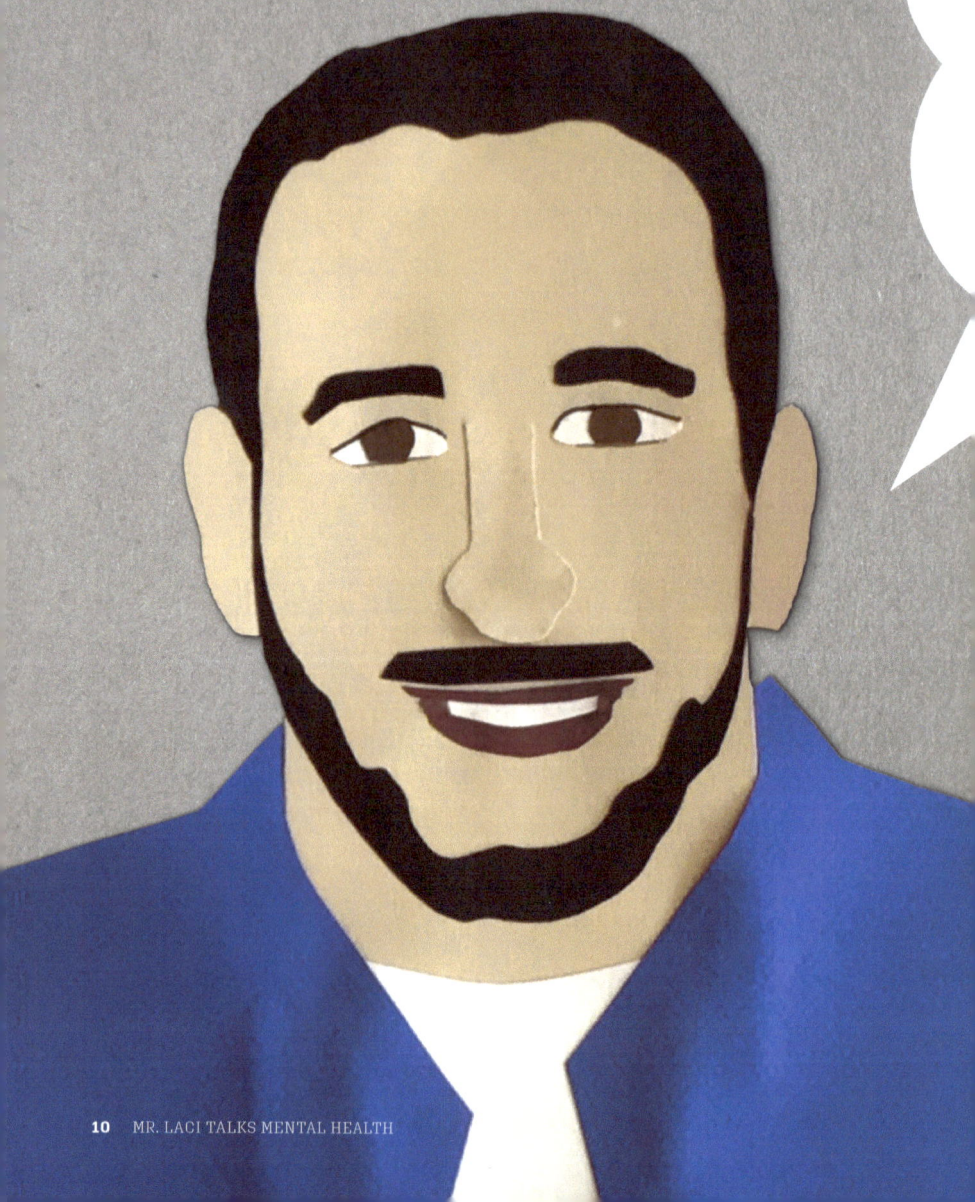

Dr. Richard Boccio Says

"We all have physical health. We go to the doctor or dentist for help with our body and teeth. We also have mental health, and we see another kind of doctor or specialist who helps people with their emotional well-being."

"Mental health can be described as our psychological health and affects how we feel, think, and act each day. It is normal to feel a variety of emotions as there are many experiences in our lives that we respond to. However, if you feel unusually anxious, worried, afraid, depressed, angry, or uneasy, you may need help in sorting out your emotions."

"You may also want to talk to a specialist if you notice any changes with your energy level, sleep schedule, or find you are eating more or less than usual. These can be physical signs of mental health challenges."

"If you feel there is a problem with your mental health, do not worry. Mental health difficulties are common and there are a lot of ways to fully recover. Talk to an adult or professional with whom you are comfortable. They want to help."

"I would also like to encourage you to pay attention to your senses. When we use our five senses, it allows us to focus on what is around us. As depression narrows our focus, expanding our view using our senses helps us appreciate the world we live in. Step outside to smell, touch, taste, listen, and look at your surroundings. This simple exercise will help you relax. Take a moment and enjoy!"

Social Distancing

It is normal to have both good days and bad days. If you are practicing social distancing, bad days are natural to experience. This is especially true in the beginning of a transition going from normal, everyday life, to having a more isolated schedule.

An easy way to improve your mood is by getting natural sunlight. It sounds simple, but it is incredibly effective. After applying sunscreen, do your best to get outside and enjoy 15 minutes of sunshine. The natural sunlight synthesizes Vitamin D, which can be considered a mood elevator. While enjoying natural sunlight, it is a great time to focus on each of your senses.

Deeper Dive

Signs that children are experiencing anxiety include refusing to do things or acting upset or scared. There are also symptoms that others are unable to see, including feeling nervous, worried, or afraid. Other signs include "having butterflies in their stomach," a racing heart, dry mouth, clammy hands, being short of breath, and/or feeling jittery.

To help at home, you can: schedule an appointment with a pediatrician. Encourage your child to take small steps in the right direction. Make sure your child gets daily physical activity, enough sleep, and eats nutritious meals. Be patient and create a caring relationship with your child to let them know you love, accept, and understand them. Enjoy your time together doing activities you both enjoy.

Depression is a kind of mood disorder where children are sad or irritable for anywhere from weeks, to months, and longer. With depression, it is hard for kids to make an effort, even if it is for activities they normally enjoy. Everyday problems also seem more difficult than they actually are.

Activity
TAPPING INTO OUR SENSES

L et's tap into our senses by using short phrases and descriptive words to answer the following questions. Afterwards, create a poem with your answers.

1. Where is your favorite place to go?

2. What do you see?

3. What sounds or noises do you hear?

4. What scents or odors do you smell?

5. What are you doing at this location?

6. Who is with you?

7. How does this make you feel?

Day 2

SELF-EXPRESSION AND GRATITUDE

with

Ms. Chris Helene Bridge

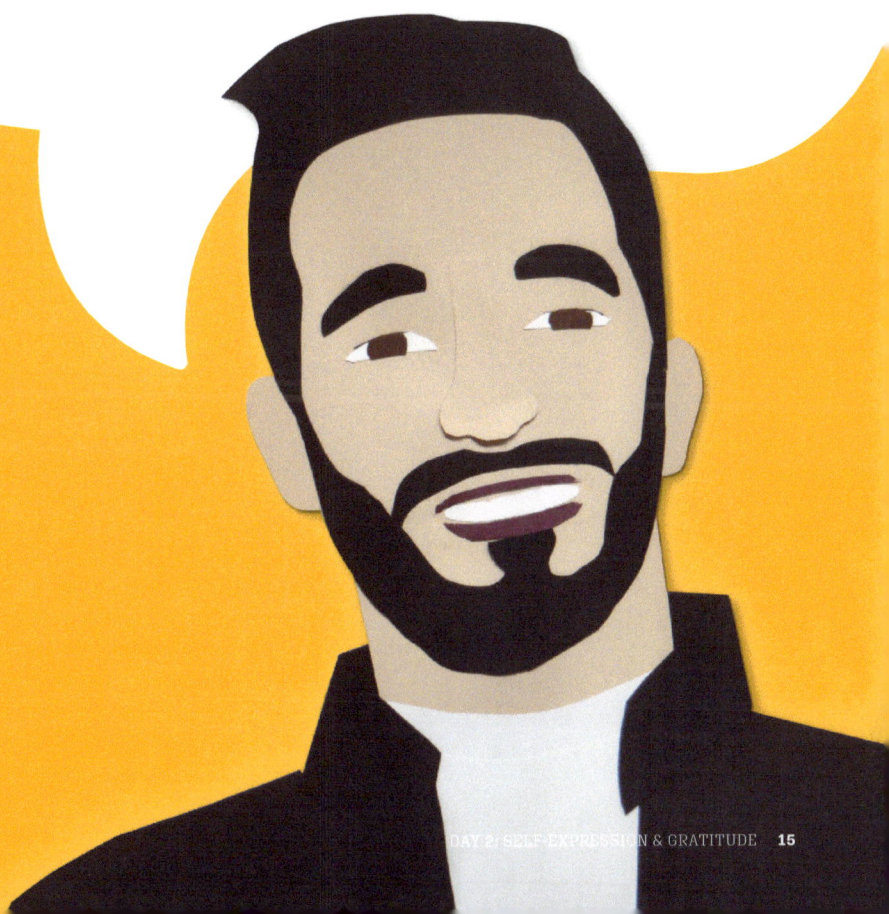

Mr. Lanci Says

1. We are all unique

2. Be creative

3. Express gratitude

Meet the Expert

Ms. Chris Helene Bridge is an award-winning author, artist, and literacy advocate from Houston, Texas. Her creative work continues to make a difference to people worldwide.

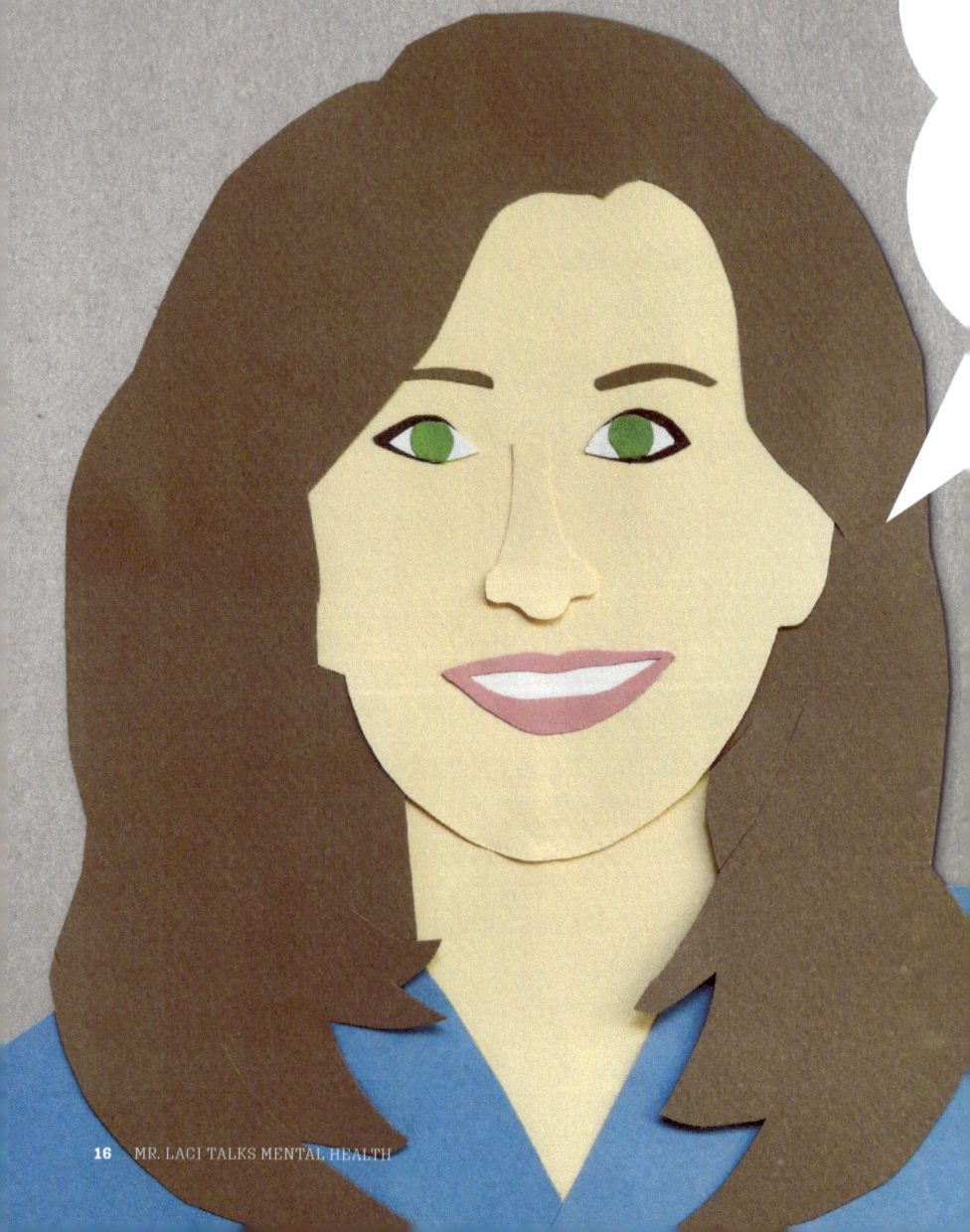

Ms. Chris Helene Bridge Says

"Both self-expression and gratitude are two vital ways to improve our mental health."

"Each day, we have around 60,000 thoughts. If we are having thoughts we do not want to have, being creative can transform our mood."

"Everyone is a creator. What makes us unique is that we all use different mediums with which we create. Some draw, paint, or write. Others cook, create music, or dance. Still others create with numbers, explore new ideas, make plans, or invent."

"Engaging in creative activities can help calm your body and brain, similar to meditation. When we create, there is often a ripple effect. The joyful energy first experienced by the creator spreads to others who experience the results of their creation. Sharing our creative interests and talents through whatever we make brings satisfaction and purpose to our lives and is a gift to others."

"Gratitude is another important aspect of mental health. Being grateful leads to less anxiety, depression, and stress, while also increasing happiness. Genuine gratitude is also linked to improved quality of sleep, which in turn, improves our mood. The more you slow down and appreciate the things in your life, the more you will find in your life to appreciate! Make a habit of counting your blessings every day!"

Social Distancing

The wonderful part about creativity is you are in charge of how you engage in it. If you are practicing social distancing, it is a great chance for you to think outside of the box about something you are passionate about or to try something new.

If you need to collaborate with or seek advice from someone else, utilizing the video chat feature on your phone or computer is a great option.

Creating a daily gratitude journal is a great activity when practicing social distancing. You may find it changes your perspective and improves your life!

Deeper Dive

When children act creatively, they are nurturing their emotional health and fostering their mental health by providing opportunities for new ways of thinking, problem solving, and trying out new ideas. Creativity acknowledges the uniqueness in children.

It is important to express genuine appreciation and gratitude for specific things you already have in your life. It is a great practice to learn to not think like a victim who wishes they had or deserve more of something.

Activity
GRATITUDE & ACHIEVEMENT LOG

Include two things you are grateful for and two things you accomplish each day for one week.

	Grateful	Accomplished
Sunday		
Monday		
Tuesday		
Wednesday		
Thursday		
Friday		
Saturday		

Day **3**

LIVING A
HEALTHY
LIFESTYLE

with

Mr. Jon Infeld

Mr. Lanci Says

1. Exercise
2. Eat healthy
3. Stay hydrated

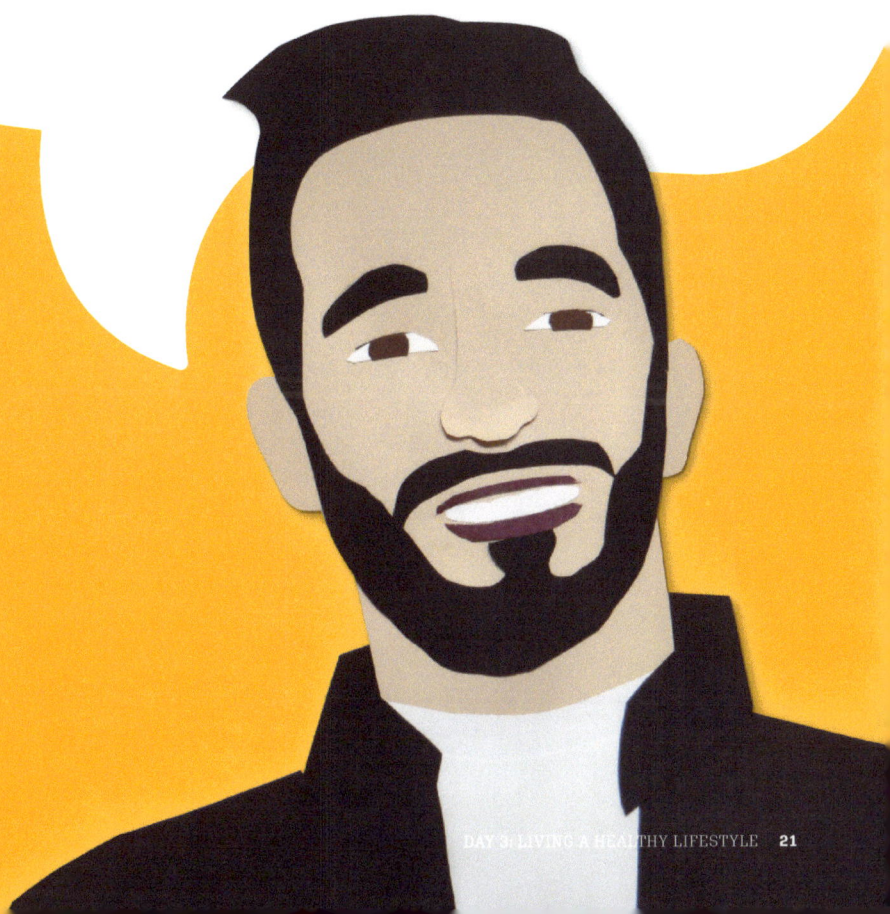

Meet the Expert

Mr. Jon Infeld is a Health and Physical Education Teacher in New Jersey. Growing up a student-athlete and being a Traumatic Brain Injury (TBI) survivor, Infeld is committed to helping others achieve optimal health.

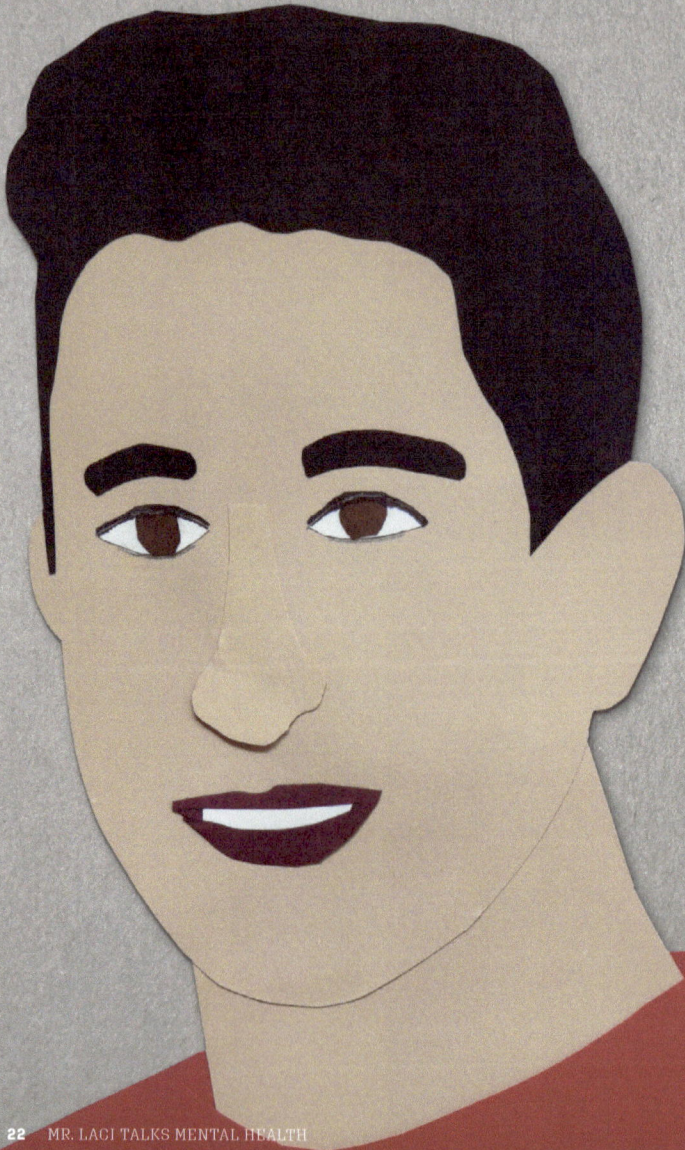

Mr. Jon Infeld Says

"Everyone understands that exercising has benefits for your physical health, but the benefits it has for your mental health are equally important for you."

"The mental benefits from exercising include improved self-esteem, reduced anxiety and stress, increased energy levels, and a lifted mood. Exercising does not mean only lifting weights, but also can include walking and less-strenuous activities."

"The foods we eat affect our feelings, moods, and cognitive function. If your diet is filled with whole grains, fresh fruits, vegetables, and lean proteins, it can help improve your general feelings of happiness and overall mood. It also reduces symptoms of depression."

"Consuming sugars may increase the likelihood you develop depression, affect your mood, and/or decrease your ability to handle stress. Also, withdrawing from a sweets-filled diet may mimic a panic attack."

"Each system in our body relies on water, and this includes our brain. Around 75% of brain tissue is water. Dehydration causes our brains to function slower and has been linked to anxiety and depression. Depending on stress levels, climate, weight, gender, and exercise levels, your daily water intake may vary. It is important to drink water throughout the day."

"Signs of dehydration include dry skin, feeling tired, dry mouth, dizziness, and dark-colored urine, among others. Drinking alcohol may also cause dehydration, along with sleep disruption and many other negative effects for your mental health."

Social Distancing

The ability to exercise does not change when you are practicing social distancing. If you thrive from the energy of others, a valuable option may be to utilize the video chat feature on your phone or computer while exercising.

If you are practicing social distancing, buying groceries is a great way to dedicate yourself to eating healthier choices. Get creative with the meals you cook. As we learned from Ms. Bridge, creativity is excellent for our overall mental health.

If you are practicing social distancing, life has slowed down and it may become difficult to remember to drink enough water. When your daily schedule is altered, a helpful tool to remind yourself to stay hydrated can be setting reminders or alerts on your phone, computer, or watch.

Deeper Dive

Mr. Lanci and Mr. Infeld both suffered a Traumatic Brain Injury (TBI) and now do their part to create mental health awareness. A TBI is when an injury causes damage to your brain and changes the way your brain works.

Similar to children, adults can suffer from ADHD (Attention Deficit Hyperactivity Disorder), too. One way to treat ADHD without a prescription is exercise. When you exercise, your brain releases chemicals. One chemical is dopamine, which helps with clearer thinking. Those with ADHD normally have less dopamine than usual in their brain.

Talk to your children's school Phys-Ed teacher to learn about exercises you can do together. Junk food commercials and peer pressure can make it difficult to ensure your child is eating healthy when you are not around. It is important to make sure your child has whole, minimally processed foods. It is rare for dehydration to cause anxiety or depression by itself, but failing to drink an adequate amount of water can put an individual at risk for increased symptoms.

Activity
CREATIVITY & FITNESS

You have now heard from both Ms. Bridge & Mr. Infeld. Let's get *creative* with *fitness* choices and healthy *eating*. For one week, challenge yourself to engage in any form of physical activity for at least 30 minutes with some healthy food to follow.

Track your progress. If you enjoy how you feel after one week, turn it into a lifestyle.

	Type of exercise	Number of minutes
Sunday		
Monday		
Tuesday		
Wednesday		
Thursday		
Friday		
Saturday		

Day 4

LOVE AND CARE

with

Dr. Denise McDermott

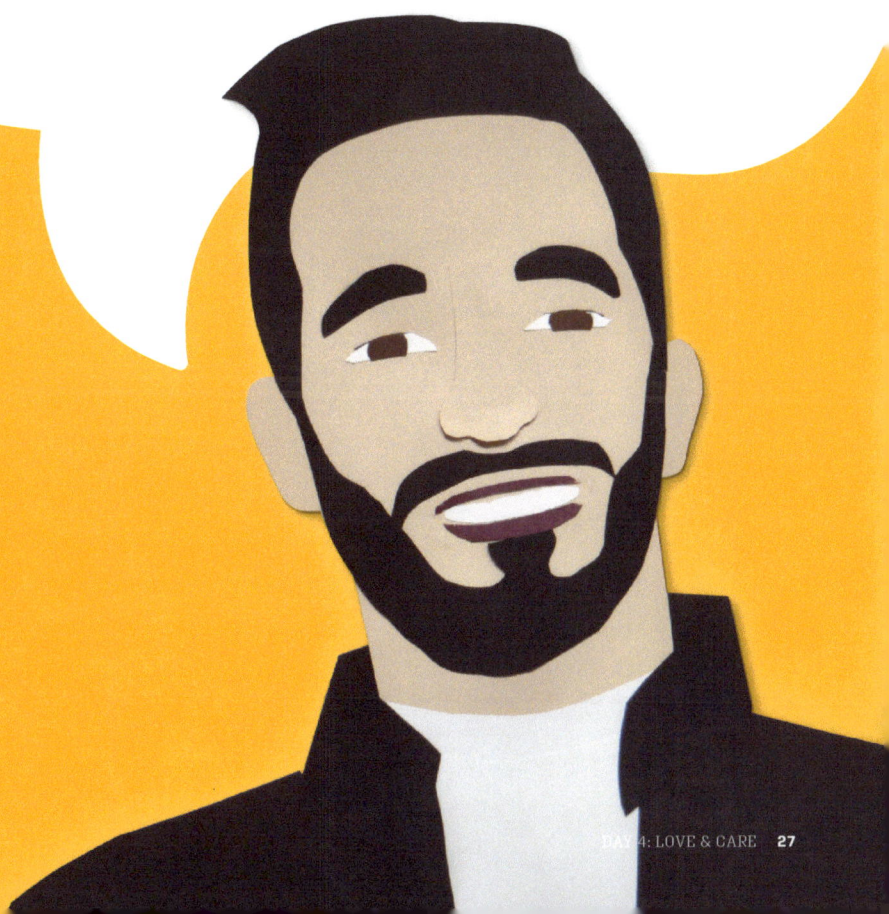

Mr. Lanci Says

1. Love and care for yourself

2. It is okay to have feelings and emotions

3. It is okay to talk to somebody

Meet the Expert

Dr. Denise McDermott, M.D. has been in private practice since 2001 as a medical doctor with board certifications in both Adult and Child Psychiatry. Her goal is to empower you, your child, and your family to live the best life possible. Her approach is to encourage people to believe in wellness, not illness, and to lead a balanced healthy lifestyle.

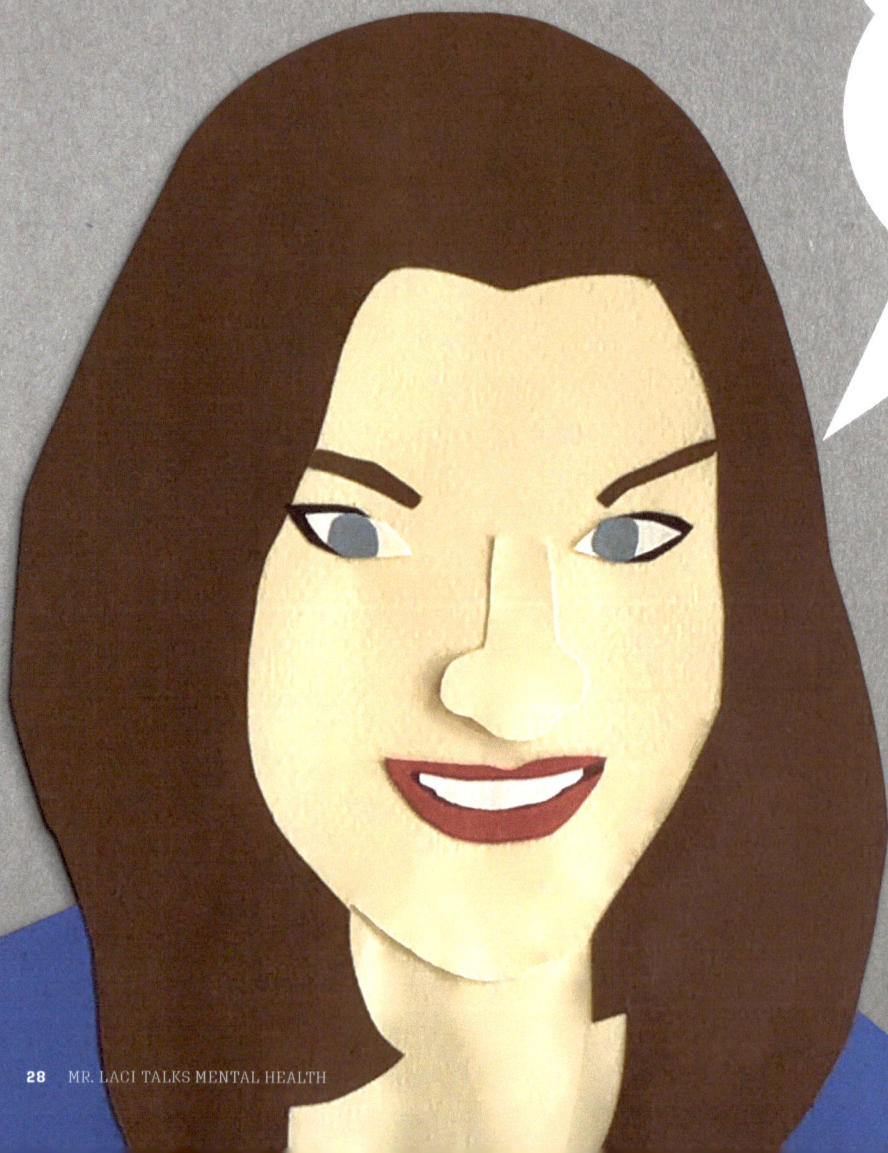

Dr. Denise McDermott Says

"Many know me around the world as "Dr. Denise." As an Adult and Child Psychiatrist, one of my most important missions is breaking the stigma associated with mental health. A psychiatrist is a medical doctor who focuses on mental health. Sometimes people come to see me when they are sad. Other times, people come to see me to stay happy. Remember, even if we are having a bad moment or experience, we can shift our feelings and have a better day."

"We need to be kind to ourselves. It is important to talk nicely to ourselves and find inner peace. The power of words and thoughts can make us feel well or unwell. Life can become busy but is important to not forget about *you*. Practice self-care and self-love by doing things you are truly passionate about."

"You are your own healer. People often look outside for the answers. Many look at their teachers, parents, and friends, but you need to find your own inner peace and be your own best friend, too. We need to tell ourselves things that are kind and that calm us down, not make us anxious."

"I am going to introduce you to a word I invented called *Neurostyle™*. We all have a *Neurostyle™*. A *Neurostyle™* is a combination of everything we are. We can drop the *Neuro*, and we all have our own *Style!* Mine is that I like to achieve and help others."

"Find and embrace your *Neurostyle™*."

Social Distancing

2020 was a year that shifted the way the world works. The *2020 COVID-19 Pandemic* was very traumatic for most individuals, especially those battling mental illnesses.

If you need to speak with a professional while you are social distancing, help is readily available. By utilizing the video chat feature on your phone or computer, you are able to speak with a psychiatrist if needed. A commonly used company is *Teladoc*.

Deeper Dive

Psychiatrists often prescribe medications in combination with psychotherapy. They are able to assess both the mental and physical aspects of psychological problems.

If you feel as if something is not normal, or the results from *2020 COVID-19 Pandemic* are still very difficult to manage, do not hesitate to speak with a professional.

Activity
CREATE YOUR NEUROSTYLE

A *Neurostyle™* is an all-encompassing word that can be used to talk about every individual's unique way of perceiving the world. As humans, we all process and perceive information in our own, unique way; biological, psychological, social, spiritual, and cultural. *Neurostyle™* does not discriminate on race, age, or gender. We process and perceive information in our own unique way.

It is time to brainstorm! Gather your thoughts with the following questions:

1. If you were having a party, would you like to invite 2 or 20 people?

2. On a typical Friday evening, would you like to stay home or go out?

3. Do you prefer the city or suburbs?

4. Would you rather cook or order your meal?

5. How do you prefer to receive your news? Written text or video?

To learn more about yourself, head to The Myers & Briggs Foundation in the ***Works Cited*** at the end of the book titled "Myers Biggs."

Day 5

YOGA, MEDITATION, AND SPIRITUALITY

with
Mr. Tony Alexander

Mr. Lanci Says

1. Practice yoga
2. Meditate
3. Spirituality

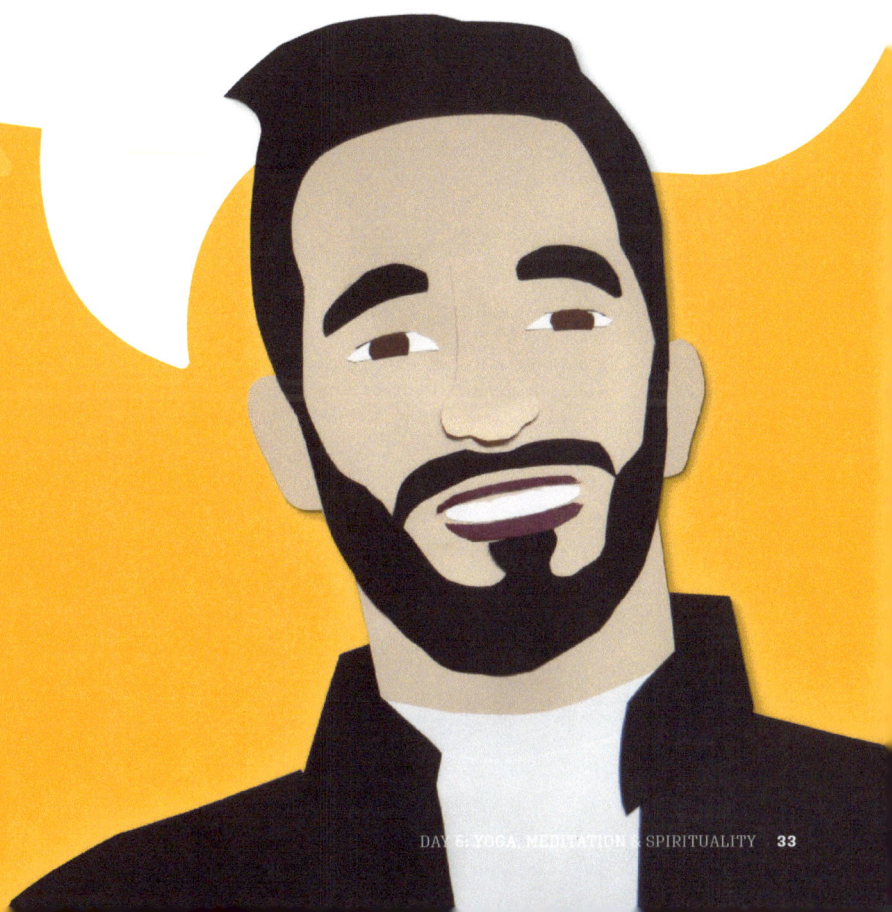

Meet the Expert

Mr. Tony Alexander is a Mental Health Advocate from Houston, Texas. He uses his voice to raise awareness for mental health and assists people in better understanding the basics about their emotions and feelings.

Alexander uses his personal experiences and leadership abilities to bring people together, while also advocating for diversity and inclusion.

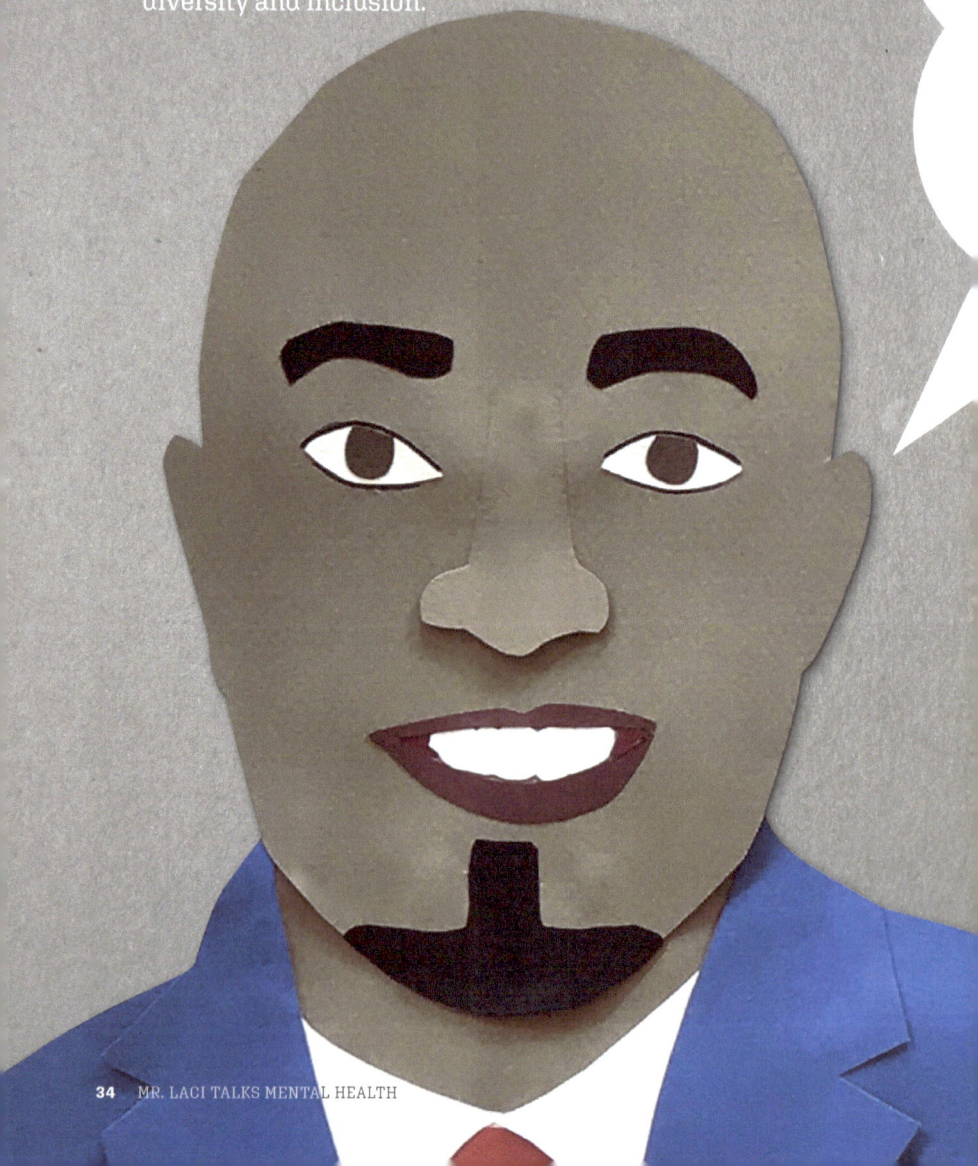

Mr. Tony Alexander Says

"I have been advocating for mental health awareness for as long as I can remember. When I was growing up, I began exercising and lifting weights because information on its benefits became readily available. Now, the same can be said for practicing activities such as yoga, meditation, and spirituality."

"Meditation can be defined as the act of giving your attention to only one thing. Practicing meditation has several amazing benefits for our mental health. It gives us the opportunity to unplug when we become overwhelmed or stressed. Meditating also improves our sleep, breathing, and focus. Practicing meditation is very beneficial for people struggling with anxiety."

"Yoga can be described as a relaxing form of exercise that involves holding postures that stretch the limbs and muscles, doing breathing exercises, and using meditation techniques to calm the mind. Many have experienced a "fight-or-flight" feeling. Yoga can help reduce this emotion. Practicing yoga helps move our nervous system from the sympathetic nervous system to parasympathetic. Put more simply, from "fight-or-flight" to "rest-and-digest." Additionally, performing yoga exercises help boost confidence and mindfulness, while also reducing stress."

"We have touched on our body and mind, but I would like to also talk about our spirituality. Integrating spirituality creates purpose, peace, and forgiveness and helps an individual tolerate stress. It is connecting to something much larger than ourselves and helps people find their interpretation of the meaning of life. Utilizing your body, mind, and spirit will elevate your mental health to new levels."

Social Distancing

If you are practicing social distancing, meditation and yoga are well-suited options to better your mental health. You do not need anyone else to perform these exercises. In fact, many choose to work on these techniques by themselves after learning the proper education. These two techniques are of no cost and provide a tremendous value to your mind.

Whether you choose to practice these methods indoors or outdoors, the choice is yours. As you learned earlier, natural sunlight is extremely beneficial for you. By combining that with yoga, you are doing a wonderful service for your brain.

Spirituality is similar in that it can be practiced wherever you feel most comfortable. To think about the best location to practice, think somewhere with a beautiful surrounding to appreciate your connection with the natural environment.

Deeper Dive

These are great activities to join in with your kids. Giving your children the tool of meditation will encourage healthy habits throughout their lives. It will also create a basic coping mechanism if he or she should experience trauma, pain, or other challenges throughout their lives.

Adults engaging in romantic relationships will find yoga to be beneficial, as when one becomes peaceful with themselves, it allows them to view their partner the same way. Spirituality helps adults when they are looking to grow, as it allows an individual to look within themselves to gain understanding on how to do so.

Children become overwhelmed and stressed, just as adults do. There is a chance children exhibit more stress than adults, but do not understand the proper coping mechanisms or language to battle their struggles.

A great link for beginners with Meditation can be found on page 51 on the **Works Cited** page titled "Meditation for Beginners."

Activity
WHAT CAN WE LEARN?

Although using applications on a smartphone are effective, meditating can also be done without an app. Here is a simple way to get started. Let's begin!

1. Get comfortable
   I. Choose a location where you feel relaxed. This can be indoors or outdoors.
   II. Prepare yourself to sit still for a few minutes.

2. Focus on your breathing
   I. Where do you notice you are breathing the most? Perhaps your nose? In your stomach?
   II. Pay attention to your inhaling and exhaling.

3. Follow your breathing
   I. For two minutes, follow your breath.
   II. Enjoy a deep inhale, which expands your stomach, and then exhale very slowly with the goal to elongate the exhale as your stomach contracts.

Source: https://www.mindful.org/how-to-meditate

Day 6

SOCIALIZING AND SUPPORT

with

Mr. James Durand

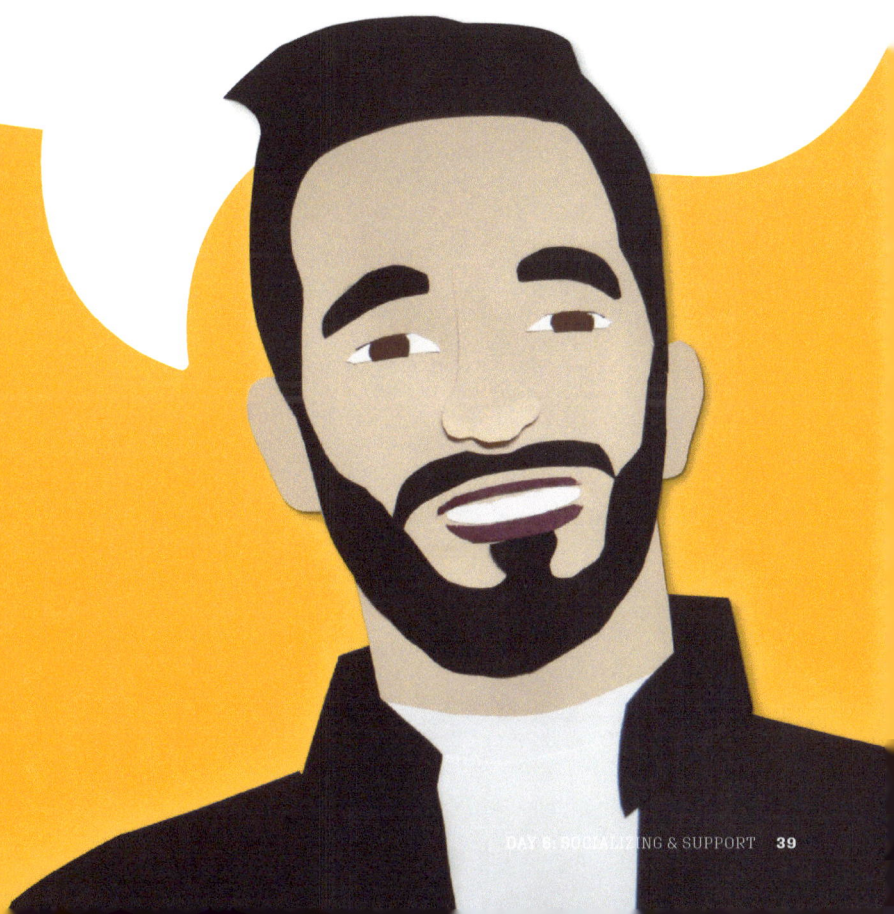

Mr. Lanci Says

1. Socialize

2. Be supportive for others

3. Be supportive of yourself

Meet the Expert

Mr. James Durand is an elementary school counselor in New York. He strives to make the lives of his students more whole. After graduating from Stony Brook University, he continued to study MSSW, Master of Science in Social Work, at Columbia University.

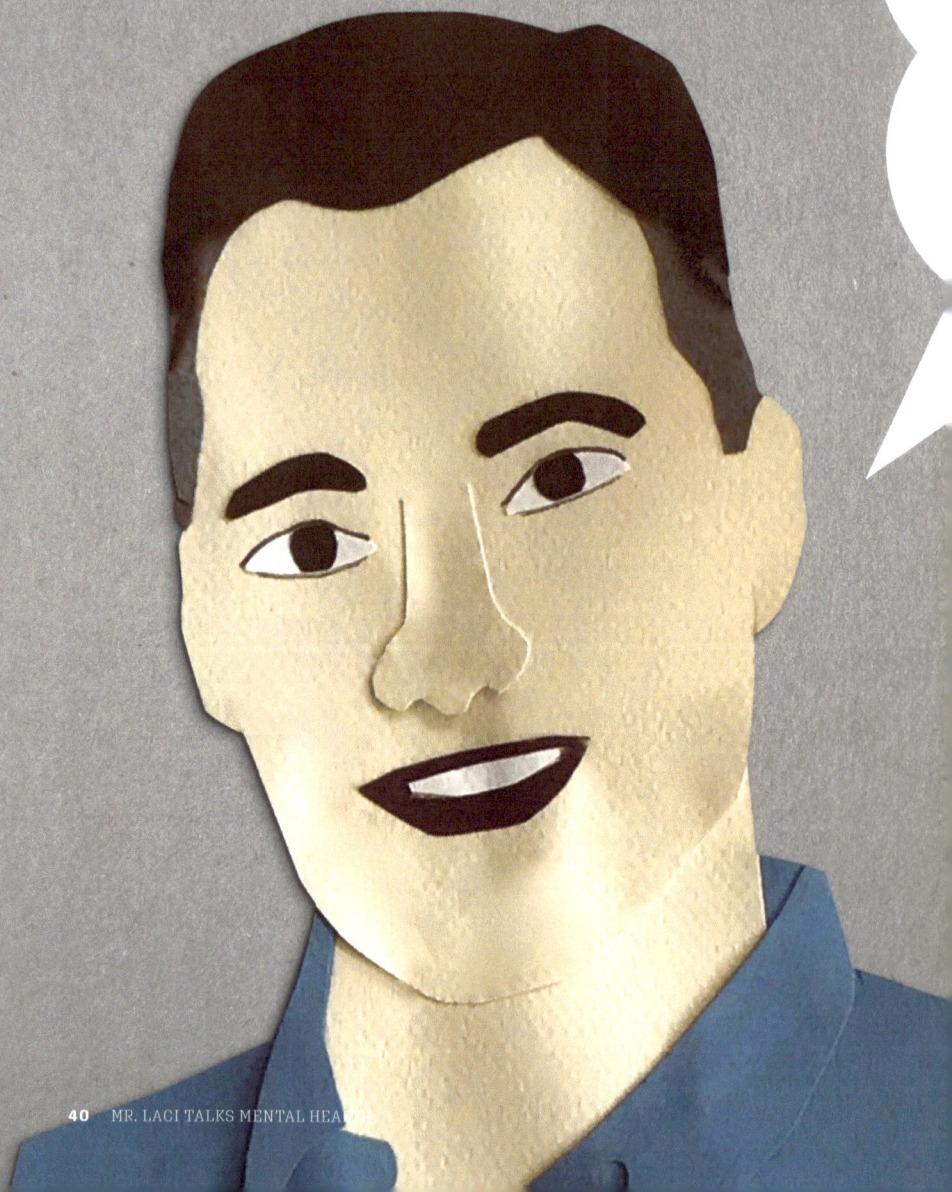

Mr. Durand Says

"Interacting with others makes us happier and improves our mood. It is an amazing way to feel better when things are not going well. Social interactions provide you with a feeling of relatedness and allow you to share your experiences to feel part of a group. It lowers the chances of feeling depressed and alone."

"Talking with others is one way we support each other. Having a support group can be very helpful when life gets challenging. This can include friends or family who you can talk to about the good and bad times in life."

"Just as we need to be supportive for others, we also need to be supportive of ourselves. As "Dr. Denise" taught us, we need to practice self-care and self-love. Additionally, I would like to recommend practicing self-compassion. By practicing this, you are creating the ability for yourself to both recognize when times are difficult and to release judgements on yourself."

"Many of you have heard of the terms independence and codependence. There is also something called interdependence. Interdependence is what we should strive for. It is the healthy balance in relationships that connect us to others, where people both give and receive support."

"An example of interdependence can be a close personal relationship, like two best friends who are supportive of each other."

Social Distancing

You never know what people are going through on any given day. Those in your inner circle may be counting on you, and the transition into social distancing may be more difficult for others than yourself.

When practicing social distancing, we can video chat our friends on our computers and phones. It will create an organic feeling as if both parties are in the same room and allow you to smile together. Check in on your friends. As Mr. Alexander says, make sure to give your friends and family, *"A Checkup From the Neck Up!"*

Deeper Dive

A great activity for you and your children can be to set up a game night with your children's friends and their parents. Teaching your children to feel comfortable socializing will provide benefits throughout many situations they will face later in life.

With social distancing protocols in effect, Margaret Mahler's "Separation-Individuation Theory of Child Development" comes into play. Although her theory applies to younger children, the idea still applies. She introduced how infants and young children separate from their parents and become their own identity in phases.

Children begin to gain a sense of individuality and independence when they go to school. However, when situations such as the 2020 *COVID-19 Pandemic* come into play, the ability to learn and grow on their own is limited.

Mr. Durand has recommended to not be directly on top of your child at home. It may help to give your child an increasing amount of additional independence over time. This can start with letting your child work on their assignments independently before offering help.

Activity
CHECK UP FROM THE NECK UP

You have now met Mr. Alexander and Mr. Durand. Let's get creative once again and combine the ideas from the two experts.

Write down five of your closest family members or friends that you have not spoken to in some time.

Write down one thing you like about each of them, one of your favorite memories with them, and one idea for your next gathering.

1. Name:
1 Thing You Like About Them:
1 Memory:
Future Plans:

2. Name:
1 Thing You Like About Them:
1 Memory:
Future Plans:

3. Name:
1 Thing You Like About Them:
1 Memory:
Future Plans:

4. Name:
1 Thing You Like About Them:
1 Memory:
Future Plans:

5. Name:
1 Thing You Like About Them:
1 Memory:
Future Plans:

Day **7**

REST AND BREAKS

with

Mr. Vincent A. Lanci

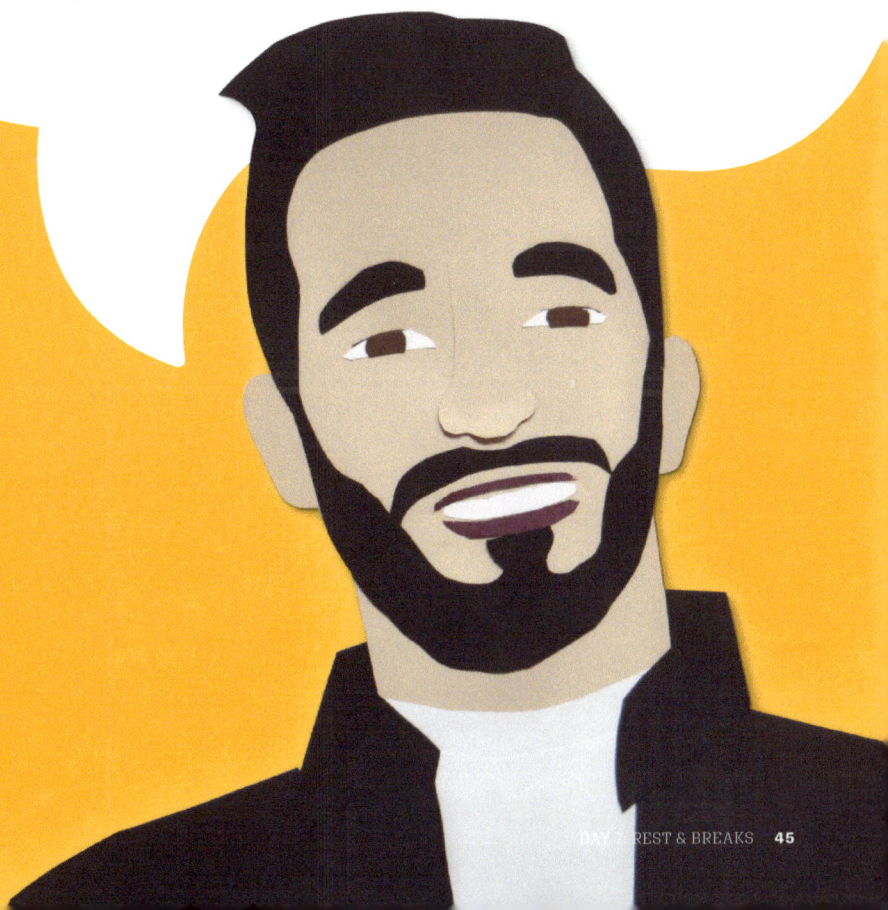

Mr. Lanci Says

1. Regularly rest both your body and mind

2. Take mental health breaks each day

3. Give yourself a mental health day each week

Meet the Expert

Vincent A. Lanci earned his MBA from The University of Tampa and currently resides in Tampa, Florida. He is an author, entrepreneur, mental health champion, and host of his podcast, *A Mental Health Break with Vincent A. Lanci*. After surviving the hit-and-run accident, he has been relentless in advocating for mental health awareness.

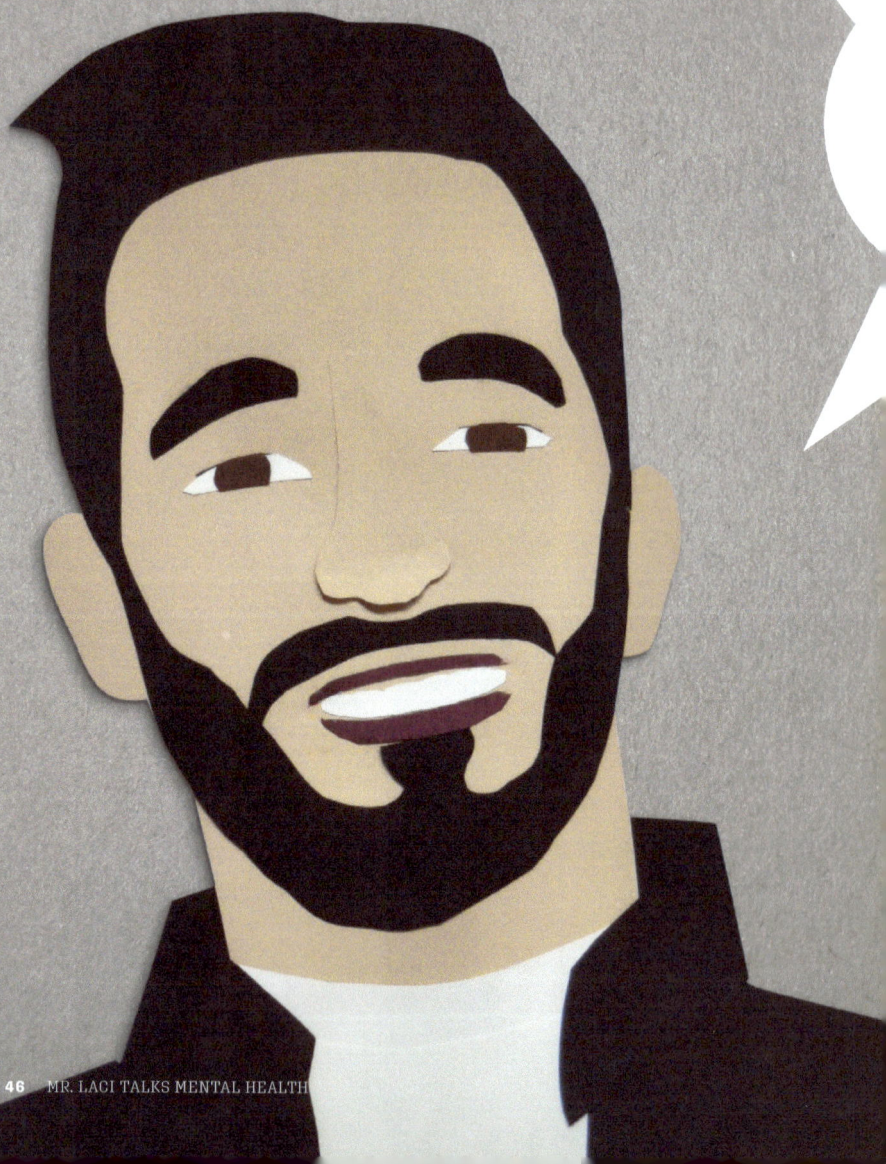

Vincent A. Lanci Says

"Mental health and sleep are very closely connected. Not getting enough sleep, or sleep deprivation, affects both your mental health and psychological state. Depression, anxiety disorders, bipolar behaviors, ADHD, among others, can be related to sleep deprivation."

"When we take a break, we can refocus and feel less stressed. Taking breaks has been shown to be crucial in recovering from stress. A relaxing break facilitates recovery by returning your physical and mental functional systems to their baseline."

"As an entrepreneur, many days exceed a 12-hour workday. A few of my most enjoyable breaks include exercising, cooking, and spending time in nature."

"Taking a mental health day is not only very important for adults, but kids, too. As humans, we need to rest our brains and bodies from our normal routines to stay mentally and physically healthy. For kids, that means no school or no homework. We need to take the time to enjoy our hobbies and spend time with the people who matter most to us."

"The day I choose to pursue my mental health day varies depending on my current workload and the time of year. During the fall, I choose to take my mental health day on Sunday each week. I enjoy either watching the Jets play on television or going to a game with friends and family."

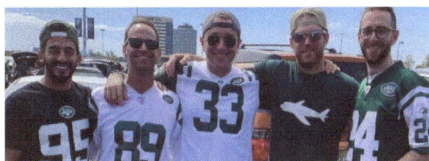

Social Distancing

It is easy to lose track of time. A good way to remember to take a break each day is to set an alarm for a certain time every hour while you are working on your obligations. Of course, many people enjoy spending time with friends and family and choose to do that on their day off or mental health day.

When practicing social distancing, make the most of your alone time. You may now have time to catch up on past interests. As we learned from "Dr. Denise," self-care and self-love are very important.

If you are practicing social distancing, you may have to change the specific details of your mental health day. You can still spend the day focusing on one of your passions. Instead of playing soccer with friends, for example, you can shoot by yourself or watch a game on TV.

Deeper Dive

Taking breaks and recovering from work-related stress can restore energy and mental resources, while decreasing the development of sleep disorders and fatigue. Emphasize taking breaks to your children when possible. When their stress decreases, you will see an increase in their performance and focus.

Making sure you and your children are not suffering from sleep deprivation is very important.

Recommended Sleep:
0-3 Months Old (Newborn): 14-17 hours • 4-11 Months Old (Infant): 12-15 hours • 1-2 Years Old (Toddler): 11-14 hours • 3-5 Years Old (Preschool): 10-13 hours • 6-13 Years Old (School-Age): 9-11 hours • 14-17 Years Old (Teenager): 8-10 hours • 18-25 Years Old (Young Adult): 7-9 hours • 26-64 Years Old (Adult): 7-9 hours • 65+ Years Old (Older Adult): 7-8 hours

Activity
TRAVEL BACK IN TIME

Travel back to a time not too long ago… a time without cell phones.

Take 30 minutes each day for one week to disconnect from the world.

Choose something you enjoy and go out and do it. Track what you do each day of the week below to reflect at week's end.

What will you do the same or different next week?

Sunday

Monday

Tuesday

Wednesday

Thursday

Friday

Saturday

How We Met

Lanci and Dr. Boccio graduated from both Northport High School and The University of Tampa together. Dr. Boccio has also been a guest on Lanci's podcast series, "A Mental Health Break with Vincent A. Lanci."

Lanci met Ms. Bridge through a mutual friend, Dr. Denise McDermott. When "Dr. Denise" found out Lanci wanted to create a new book, she thought of Bridge. Lanci and Ms. Bridge collaborated to create this book, "Mr. Lanci Talks Mental Health."

Lanci and Mr. Infeld met as students in college and became roommates. You can learn more about their relationship as it relates to mental health in the "Deeper Dive" section of his day. Infeld has also been a guest on "A Mental Health Break with Vincent A. Lanci."

Lanci met Dr. Denise through networking. After writing his book, "Left for Dead: A Story of Redemption," he reached out to Dr. Denise to send her a book in efforts to collaborate and break down mental health stigmas together. This new friendship led her to becoming the first guest on "A Mental Health Break with Vincent A. Lanci" and a later guest on Lanci's second podcast, "What It's Really Like to Be an Entrepreneur."

Lanci and Mr. Alexander met through Lanci's cousin, Kim. When Kim learned what Lanci was up to professionally, she thought the introduction would be valuable to them both. Mr. Alexander has since been a guest on "A Mental Health Break with Vincent A. Lanci."

Mr. Durand was Mr. Lanci's school counselor when he was a student at Pulaski Road Elementary School. Mr. Durand has since brought Lanci back to his old elementary school to speak as a guest on "Leadership Day."

Works Cited

1. "Anxiety Disorders," *reviewed by D'Arcy Lyness, PhD in "KidsHealth"*
   a. https://kidshealth.org/en/parents/anxiety-disorders.html#:~:text=They%20might%20act%20scared%20or,jittery%2C%20or%20short%20of%20breath.
2. "Depression," *reviewed by D'Arcy Lyness, PhD in "KidsHealth"*
   a. https://kidshealth.org/en/parents/understanding-depression.html
3. "31 Tips To Boost Your Mental Health" in "Mental Health America"
   a. https://www.mhanational.org/31-tips-boost-your-mental-health
4. "Here's How Creativity Actually Improves Your Mental Health," *contributed to by Ashley Stahl, in "Forbes"*
   a. https://www.forbes.com/sites/ashleystahl/2018/07/25/heres-how-creativity-actually-improves-your-health/#3746944713a6
5. "The Importance of Being Grateful," *by Deborah Jepsen in "Melbourne Child Psychology & School Psychology Services"*
   a. https://www.melbournechildpsychology.com.au/blog/importance-grateful/
6. "Creativity and Play: Fostering Creativity," in *PBS*
   a. https://www.pbs.org/wholechild/providers/play.html#:~:text=A%20child's%20creative%20activity%20can,of%20thinking%20and%20problem%2Dsolving.
7. "The Foods We Eat Do Affect Our Mental Health. Here's the Proof.," *in Psychology Today*
   a. https://www.psychologytoday.com/us/blog/evidence-based-living/202001/the-foods-we-eat-do-affect-our-mental-health-heres-the-proof
8. "Water, Depression, and Anxiety," *reviewed by Mary L. Gavin, MD, in "Solara Mental Health"*
   a. https://solaramentalhealth.com/can-drinking-enough-water-help-my-depression-and-anxiety/
9. "Why Exercise is Good for Your Mental Health," *by Christopher Morh, PhD, RD, in EatingWell*
   a. http://www.eatingwell.com/article/7822525/mental-benefits-of-exercise/
10. "What Is Psychiatry?," *American Psychiatric Association*
    a. https://www.psychiatry.org/patients-families/what-is-psychiatry-menu
11. www.DrDeniseMD.com
12. "Meditation Definition: What is Meditation? Take Care of the Mind," *in MindWorks*
    a. https://mindworks.org/blog/meditation-definition/
13. "Medical Definition of Yoga," *by William C. Shiel Jr., MD, FACP, FACR, in MedicineNet*
    a. https://www.medicinenet.com/script/main/art.asp?articlekey=10811
14. "The Benefits of Meditation For Kids," *Thrive Global*
    a. https://thriveglobal.com/stories/the-benefits-of-meditation-for-kids/
15. "5 Ways Yoga Benefits Your Mental Health," *by Jennifer D'Angelo Friedman, in Yoga Journal*
    a. https://www.yogajournal.com/lifestyle/5-ways-yoga-is-good-for-your-mental-health
16. Margaret Mahler (1897-1985), *in GoodTherapy*
    a. https://www.goodtherapy.org/famous-psychologists/margaret-mahler.html
17. "Sleep and mental health: Sleep deprivation can affect your mental health," *in Harvard Health Publishing: Harvard Medical School*
    a. https://www.health.harvard.edu/newsletter_article/sleep-and-mental-health
18. "The Importance of Taking Breaks," *in "The Well Being Thesis"*
    a. https://thewellbeingthesis.org.uk/foundations-for-success/importance-of-taking-breaks-and-having-other-interests/#:~:text=Taking%20breaks%20has%20been%20shown,and%20cardiovascular%20disease%20%5B2%5D.
19. "Severe Traumatic Brain Injury Factsheet (for Schools)" *reviewed by Mary L. Gavin, MD in "KidsHealth"*
    a. https://kidshealth.org/en/parents/tbi-factsheet.html#:~:text=A%20severe%20traumatic%20brain%20injury,temporary%20effect%20on%20brain%20function.

20. "Adult ADHD and Exercise," *in WebMD*
    a. https://www.webmd.com/add-adhd/
       adult-adhd-and-exercise
21. "Healthy Foods for Kids," *Jeanne Segal
    Ph.D & Lawrence Robinson in "HelpGuide"*
    a. https://www.helpguide.org/articles/
       healthy-eating/healthy-food-for-kids.htm
22. How Much Sleep Do We Really Need?, *in
    Sleep Foundation*
    a. https://www.sleepfoundation.org/
       articles/how-much-sleep-do-we-
       really-need
23. "The Five Senses," *in MentalHealth.net:
    An American Addiction Centers Resource*
    a. https://www.mentalhelp.net/
       depression/the-five-senses/
24. "Myers Briggs"
    a. https://www.myersbriggs.org/
       my-mbti-personality-type/mbti-basics/
25. "The Mental Health Benefits of Religion
    and Spirtuality," *in NAMI*
    a. https://www.nami.org/Blogs/NAMI-
       Blog/December-2016/The-Mental-
       Health-Benefits-of-Religion-Spiritual
26. "Depression," *in Medline Plus*
    a. https://medlineplus.gov/
       dehydration.html
27. "6 Tips for Teaching Yoga To Beginners,"
    in Yoga National
    a. https://yogainternational.com/
       article/view/6-tips-for-teaching-yoga-
       to-beginners
28. "Meditation for Beginners," *in Headspace.*
    https://www.headspace.com/meditation/
    meditation-for-beginners
29. "Teladoc"
    a. https://www.teladoc.com/
30. Your Anxiety Loves Sugar. Eat These 3
    Things Instead"
    a. https://www.healthline.com/health/
       mental-health/how-sugar-harms-
       mental-health#withdrawal
31. "Alcohol and Mental Health, *in
    MentalHealth.Org*
    a. https://www.mentalhealth.org.
       uk/a-to-z/a/alcohol-and-mental-health
32. "How to Meditate," in *Mindful*
    a. https://www.mindful.org/
       how-to-meditate/
33. "6 Tips to Love and Support Yourself and
    Become a Happier You," by Laura Delman,
    in *Tiny Buddha*
    a. https://tinybuddha.com/blog/6-tips-
       to-love-support-yourself-become-
       happier-you/

www.ingramcontent.com/pod-product-compliance
Lightning Source LLC
Chambersburg PA
CBHW040129270326
41927CB00004B/96